Juicing Recipes

50 Refreshing Juicing Recipes for Weight Loss, Detox, and Healthy Living

Jamie Fox

©2014

Table of Contents

Check out my other Book

[Smoothie Recipes: 101 Delicious Smoothie Recipes for Weight Loss, Detox, and Energy Rejuvenation](#)

The Creator of this Wonderful Juicing Recipe Book:

My name is Jamie Fox and I've been experimenting with juicing for about a year now. I became a mother September 4th of 2013 and my son is now the light of my life. I began juicing throughout my pregnancy and have continued to drink them post pregnancy to get back to my previous weight. I decided to write a juicing recipe book because I feel I have benefited from the juicing process and feel that spreading my knowledge will help others as well. My son is at the age now where he is learning to roll over, stand up with help, and attempt to crawl. Because of this, he gets up early in the morning and needs a great deal of undivided attention throughout the day. Fresh juice recipes help me stay energized while providing my body with beneficial nutrients that aid in my weight loss journey. I believe these recipes will help you do the same! I also created a smoothie recipe book that has been an aid in my weight loss journey as well. The idea of juicing was derived from my experience with smoothies, and I feel combining both practices has been a major benefit to my body and mind more than either one did on its own!

Why should you Juice?

Juicing is one of the best things we can do for our body. 95% of the enzymes and vitamins that our bodies need are provided in the juice of fresh raw fruits and vegetables. To receive the amount of enzymes and vitamins in whole fruits and vegetables we would have to eat more than five servings of each item compared to drinking twenty ounces of fresh mixed juice. When these nutrients and vitamins are consumed in liquid form, they are absorbed quickly within the blood stream, giving us the full benefits while giving our digestive system a break from the continuous digestion process. When juicing, it is best to drink the juice mixture the same day it is pressed to prevent the loss of nutritional value. If you are unable to drink the juice mixture the same day it is pressed, storing your juice mixture in a tightly enclosed glass jar will protect the juice from losing its nutritional value as quickly as leaving it uncovered. Juicing not only provides our bodies with sufficient amounts of vitamins and nutrients, but it also promotes weight loss, increases energy level, and boosts immunity. Natural vitamins and minerals that are provided within the juices of various fruits and vegetables are more beneficial than synthetic supplements. Natural vitamins and minerals are absorbed fully within our bodies, unlike synthetic supplements. It is best to ingest fresh juices on an empty stomach because it maximizes the positive effects that these plentiful vitamins and minerals possess on the body. There are many reasons it is best to press your own fresh juice compared to purchasing bottled juices. When you press your own juice, you know exactly where it is coming from and exactly what ingredients are obtained within it. When you consume pre-made store bought juice you are unaware of the exact ingredients and do not know the exact nutritional value it obtains. Fresh pressed juice is filled with lively vitamins, minerals, and nutrients. Pre-made store bought juice is pasteurized, which means the ingredients are heated and processed, which leads to the destruction of all essential nutrients that fresh fruits and vegetables possess. One of the main reasons we should all juice is because simply, it is easy! Providing your body with all its essential nutrients in one daily drink is amazing! There is no need to spend all day worrying about ingesting the proper amount of vitamins and minerals within the food we eat. Instead, prepare a delicious chill juice drink once a day and all your troubles are gone. It is also easy on our body. Drinking essential nutrients instead of eating fruits and vegetables that obtain essential nutrients gives our digestive tract a break, leading to weight loss and increased energy.

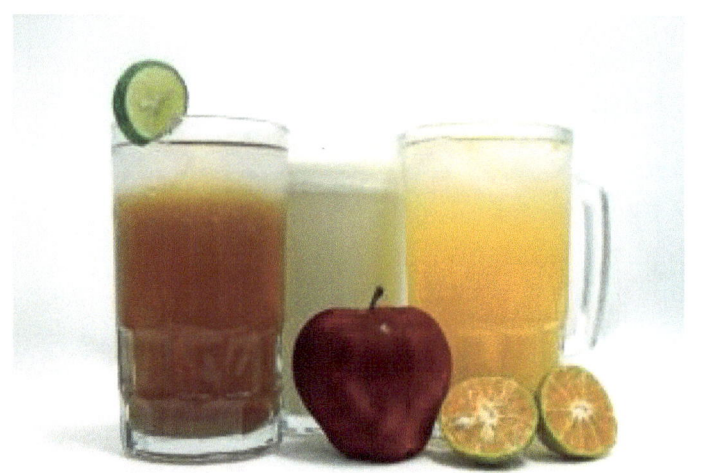

What type of juicer is best for you?

A juicer separates the nutrient filled juice from your fruits and vegetables. In reality, when we eat fruits and vegetables our digestive system does a similar process as a juicer, but in this case, juicing strongly benefits our digestive system because it does the job for us. Some juicers do better jobs than others. It all depends on how much work you are willing to do while you make your juice mixture, and how serious you are about juicing. There is no need to go buy a $300 juicer if you plan to use it a handful of times. If you are very serious about obtaining a juicing lifestyle, one of these extravagant juicers might be the right fit for you. Although there are many different styles of juicers, there are only two main types. There are centrifugal juicers and cold press juicers, each obtaining different benefits.

Centrifugal juicers are the cheaper of the two and the most common available in usual retail stores. These juicers pulverize fruits and vegetables against a round blade that spins quickly against a metal strainer, pushing the juice down and separating it from the pulp. These types of juicers are faster, cheaper, and easier to use. They also decrease the food preparation time as they do a great deal of the chopping for you. They do have negative aspects, as they produce less juice than cold press juicers. Centrifugal juicers also kill certain enzymes within the juice as they use heat during the fast spinning process. They are still beneficial to juicing purposes and if you are unable to purchase a cold press juicer due to the price, a centrifugal juicer will be perfect for you.

Cold Press Juicers operate at lower speeds and compress fruits and vegetables to slowly gather the juice within them. They produce more juice and better juice than centrifugal juicers, yet they do cost a great deal more. Because cold press juicers use slower spends, they obtain more nutrients and enzymes, allowing the juice mixture to last longer after pressing. This leads to less waste compared to centrifugal juicers. Cold press juicers have negative qualities other than their high buying price. When creating your juice, it takes longer for preparation because of the way the machine is set up, it requires smaller pieces to fit within the juicing press area. Cold press machines also obtain higher amounts of pulp due to the continuous squeezing of the fruits and vegetables.

When trying to decide between the two, ask yourself how long you plan to juice, and in the end how much money you will be saving with your choice. Although Centrifugal juicers are less expensive, they do not produce as much juice as cold press juicers which leads to the waste of juice within fruits and vegetables. Overtime, the cost of ingredients will add up. If you have a busy lifestyle and do not want to spend any more time on juicing than you have to, then maybe a centrifugal juicer is right for you since cold press juicers take longer preparation time. Each type of juicer has positive aspects as well as negative aspects, you just have to decide which juicer best fits your needs and your lifestyle.

Purchasing Ingredients: Organic or Non-organic?

There are many different fruits and vegetables that can be purchased non-organic, but there are also many that need to be purchased organic to receive the best nutrients without the use of pesticides during the growing process. Juicing, especially the recipes within this book, include ingredients that should be purchase organic. Yes, organic goods are slightly more expensive, but worth the extra change. Organic foods are produced through organic farming, with minimal synthetic inputs like fertilizers and pesticides. Organic foods are produced naturally without food additives or preservatives. Certain foods, due to their thin skin, are recommended for organic purchasing. Some foods can be bought non-organic due to their thick skin. Below are foods recommended for organic purchase and foods that can be purchased non organic. I have only included ingredients that are obtained within the juicing recipes within this book.

Recommended for Organic purchase:

-Celery

-Apples

-Strawberries

-Spinach

-Blueberries

-Lettuce/Kale

-Grapes

-Bell Peppers

-Beets

-Carrots

-Cucumbers

-Tomatoes

Foods that can be purchased Non-organic:

-Pineapple

-Avocado

-Mango

-Cantaloupe

-Kiwi

-Sweet potatoes

-Grapefruit

-Limes, Lemons

What are the Benefits of Juicing?

There are numerous benefits to the process of juicing, especially the nutrients it provides your body. The juices within fruits and vegetables are enriched with the vitamins, minerals, and nutrients that our bodies strive for. It is more convenient and more realistic to drink one large glass of numerous food juices mixed together instead of attempting to eat ten or more different foods in one day to achieve the same health benefits. Juicing gives your digestive system a break while rushing nutrients to all parts of your body that needs them. Juicing helps our bodies regulate a normal and healthy pH level, reducing our chances of obtaining an acidic imbalance that leads to health issues. Fruit and vegetable juice can help protect against cancers, inflammatory diseases, heart disease, and various bone and tissue disorders. Juicing also boosts the immune system, provides your body with nutrients resulting in increased energy, and aids weight loss. Each ingredient has its own personal benefits, which will be discussed within each section within this juicing recipe bible!

Although juicing is very beneficial to the body, please note that juicing is not a replacement for meals, whole foods, or the intake of fruits and vegetables. Juicing is a part time program as you are recommended to intake whole foods and regular sized meals along with the process of juicing for best results.

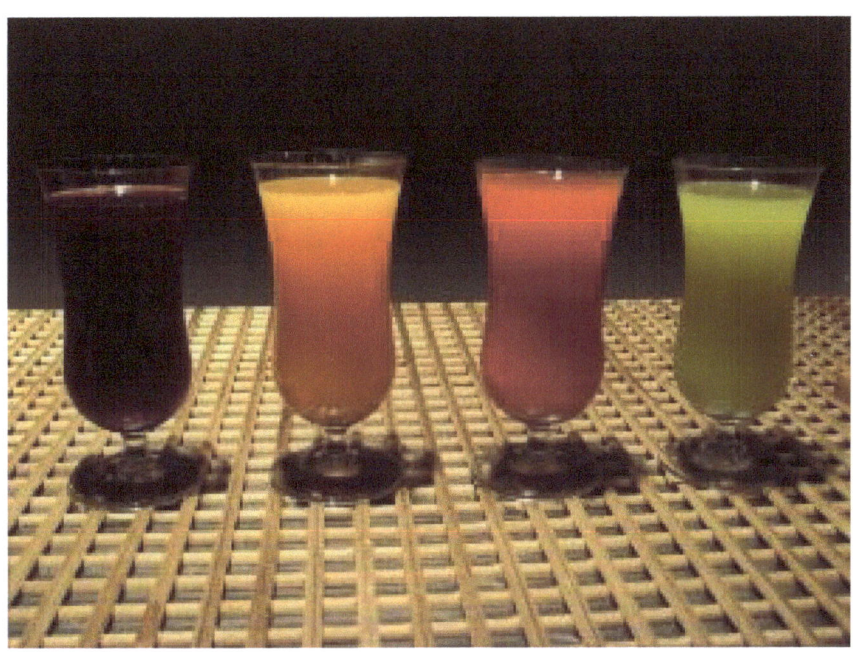

GREEN JUICING BENEFITS

There are countless body benefits for the intake of juice from green vegetables. The main benefit is in taking juice from green vegetables allows the body to receive the plentiful vitamins and minerals that are within these wonderful green vegetables. Allowing your body to receive these nutrients quicker than ingesting them as whole foods results in increased energy, better hydration, and better health. Green vegetable juice is like a natural vitamin water, providing your body with natural vitamins, minerals, nutrients, and chlorophyll that your body strives for. While some people enjoy snacking on green leafy vegetables, most individuals do not. The benefit to juicing your green veggies is you are able in intake a lot more juice that sitting down and eating these various vegetables. You are providing your body with more nutrients and minerals than you would normally from just eating these foods. Spinach, which is included in many of these recipes, provides our body with high amounts of vitamin K, B, C, and A, along with high amounts of iron, magnesium, calcium, manganese, folate, and many more. Juicing spinach extracts these various vitamins and minerals, providing your body with these nutrients in juice form without having to eat spinach as a whole food. Spinach holds antioxidant and anti-inflammatory properties unlike most green vegetables. Adding spinach to your juicing recipe ensures you are receiving excellent health benefits from one simple glass of juice!

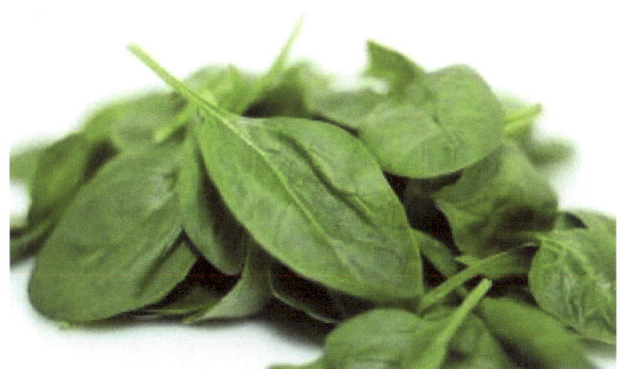

Kale, included in many of these juicing recipes, is a green leafy vegetable that is known as one of the healthiest vegetables in the world. Although kale is extremely healthy, many individuals refuse to eat kale due to its taste, texture, or the amount of chewing it takes when eating it whole. Adding kale into your juicing recipes will provide you with the numerous nutrients this ingredient provides without forcing yourself to eat something you don't particularly like. Kale is extremely low in calories while providing your body with sufficient amounts of Potassium, Vitamin A, and Vitamin C. Some say eating kale on a regular basis can decrease future health issues such as cancer and heart disease. Kale also has benefits to your outer appearance, causing your hair to grow faster and provides your skin and nails with essential oils which overall improves your appearance.

Celery is another beneficial green ingredient within these green juice recipes. Celery prevents and reduces inflammation within the body, giving relief to body aches and pains. Celery obtains levels of magnesium resulting in soothing your nervous system. So if you are feeling anxious or stressed, add a stalk or two of celery to your juice to relieve your worries! Celery also reduces blood pressure, bad cholesterol levels, delays the formation of potential future cancer cells. Another great benefit is one stalk of celery is about ten calories. Adding celery to your juicing recipes adds many nutrients while keeping calorie count low!

Green Juicing Recipes

GREENY MACHINE

Two medium granny smith apples

One large soft avocado

Two stalks of celery

Twenty green grapes

One large lime

Two cups spinach

AVOCADO BLAST

One medium cucumber

One large soft avocado

One cup spinach

One large lemon

½ pear

GREEN ESCAPE

Two cups spinach

One medium cucumber

Two stalks celery

Two granny smith apples

One large pear

GREEN RUSH

Four stalks of celery

One large avocado

Two cups spinach

Two granny smith apples

One large lemon

PEAR BEAR

One large avocado

One pear

One cup fresh pineapple

Two cups spinach

One large lime

SMOOTH BREEZE

One large soft avocado

Two cups fresh pineapple

½ large pear

One medium granny smith apple

PINE DELITE

Two stalks kale

Two cups spinach

One cup fresh pineapple

One large granny smith apple

GRANNY GREEN

Two cups green grapes

½ medium cucumber

One cup spinach

One granny smith apple

One large lime

KALE CITRUS JUICE

Four stalks of celery

Two stalks kale

Two cups spinach

Three granny smith apples

Two large limes

One inch fresh ginger root

CITRUS BLAST

Five celery stalks

½ medium cucumber

One granny smith apple

Three stalks kale

One large pear

One medium lemon

One medium lime

CARROT JUICING BENEFITS

Carrot juice is sweet in taste making it easy to drink, especially when mixed with other fruit and vegetable juices. One cup of carrot juice contains about 85 calories, making it a great alternative to other juices while providing your body with numerous benefits. Carrot juice contains Vitamin A, C, E, and B vitamins. It also contains levels of potassium which is beneficial in keeping your heart and kidneys healthy and preventing various health issues such as heart disease, cancer, and even infertility. When drinking carrot juice prior to each meal, it aids in improving digestion. Because carrots contain levels of beta-carotene and lutein, it is known to improve the health of our eyes, leading to better eyesight. Carrots are a major benefit to our skin, known to improve the dryness, appearance, and even known to clear blemishes that we all struggle with. Carrots obtain antioxidant properties which flush toxins out of our bodies and overall ensure better health. Adding carrots to your juicing recipes will provide your body with many nutrients and vitamins that most individuals do not obtain during their normal daily diet.

Many of these carrot juicing recipes contain the juice of oranges, which also provides our bodies with numerous health benefits. Fresh juice from oranges contains high levels of Vitamin C which is great for our immune system and protects against immune system deficiencies. Fresh orange juice is known to lower blood pressure and bad cholesterol levels, improving the health of the heart. Fresh orange juice contains antioxidant properties which decreases the amount of damage free radicals cause on our cells. Adding fresh squeezed orange juice to your juicing recipes will add to the amount of vitamins and nutrients you are providing your body to benefit your health.

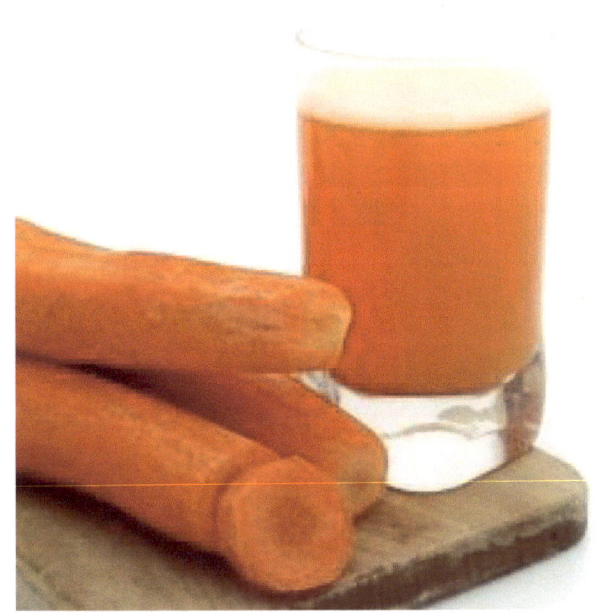

Carrot Juicing Recipes

CARROT CLEANSE

Four large carrots

½ red ruby grapefruit

1/4 teaspoon fresh chopped ginger

One medium pear

CRISP CARROT JUICE

Two stalks kale

Three large carrots

Two stalks celery

15 strawberries

One large granny smith apple

CARROT CANTALOUPE

Five large carrots

One cup fresh cantaloupe

Two stalks celery

Two large red apples

CURVY CARROT JUICE

Five large carrots

Two medium oranges

One large red apple

Two stalks celery

One cup fresh pineapple

COLORFUL CARROT JUICE

Four large carrots

One large red apple

Three stalks celery

Two stalks kale

One piece fresh ginger

CREAMY CARROT

Four large carrots

One large cucumber

Two medium oranges

One piece fresh ginger

One large red apple

CITRUS CARROT JUICE

Five large carrots

Two cups fresh mango

Two medium oranges

One piece fresh ginger

CANDID CARROT CLEANSE

Four large carrots

One large lemon

Two medium oranges

Two stalks celery

One piece fresh ginger

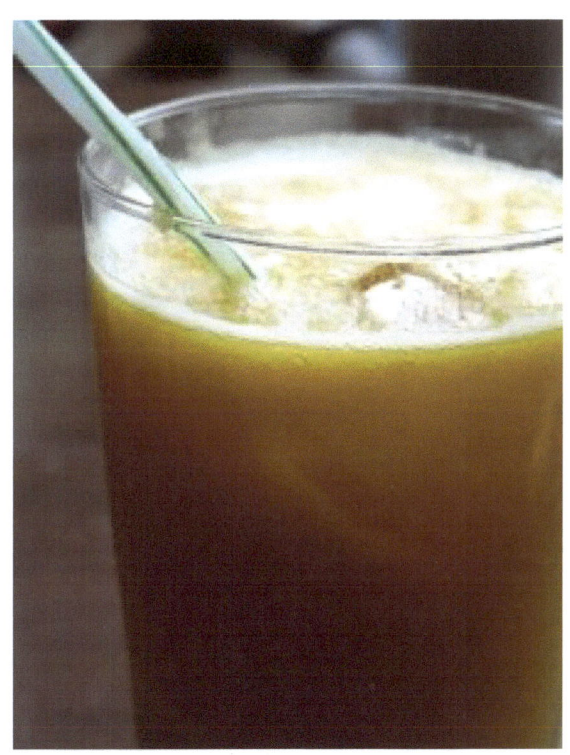

CALM CARROT

Seven large carrots

One red ruby grapefruit

Two large oranges

One small piece fresh ginger

CATCHY CARROT CLEANSE

Six large carrots

One cup fresh pineapple

Two medium oranges

One large red apple

BEET JUICING BENEFITS

Many individuals don't choose beets as their first choice for eating whole food vegetables. That is why juicing beets is an amazing way to receive the health benefits of beets without having to force yourself to get past the distinct flavor that beets possess. Beets are sweet in flavor, but they do obtain a unique taste that many individuals don't necessarily care for. Juicing beets and mixing them with other juiced fruits or vegetables will make a delicious drink with countless vitamins, minerals, and nutrients that your body strives for! Beets have been known as a liver-protecting food for many years, but recent research shows beet juice has a lot more benefits that recognized in the past. Beet juice contains many antioxidant properties and natural nitrates, which helps blood flow throughout the body. This means more blood is flowing to the brain, heart, and muscles, benefiting our bodies on a more in depth level than many other fruits and vegetables. These nitrates open blood vessels and allow more oxygen to flow within the blood throughout our bodies. Beet juice is also known to lower blood pressure, relieving uncomfortable feelings of stress and anxiety. Understand that drinking beet juice can alter the color of your urine or bowel movements, so do not be alarmed if this occurs. There are numerous benefits to the power of beet juice that everyone needs to take advantage of to live the healthiest life possible.

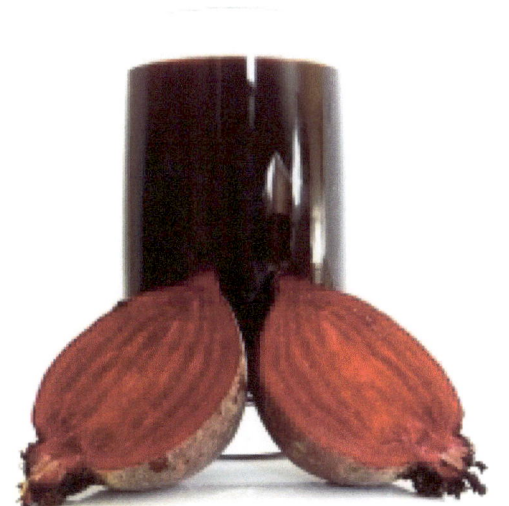

Beet Juicing Recipes

BEET EXPLOSION

One small beet chopped

Four large carrots

One granny smith apple

One large lemon

PURPLE CITRUS

One small beet chopped

Three large carrots

Two medium oranges

One large granny smith apple

RED RUBY

Two small beets chopped

Two large red apples

One large orange

One piece fresh ginger

PURPLE BERRY BEET

One red apple

One cucumber

One small beet chopped

One cup fresh blueberries

CITRUS BLEND

One small beet chopped

One lemon

Two stalks kale

Two medium oranges

One large red apple

ORANGE KICK

One beet chopped

Two large carrots

One large red apple

Two large oranges

RELAXATION MELODY

One beet

One cup spinach

One large red apple

One large lime

One medium cucumber

One piece fresh ginger

REFRESH AND REJUVENATE

One large cucumber

Two granny smith apples

One beet chopped

Three stalks kale

CARROT BEET

One beet

Five large carrots

One large orange

One large lemon

REFRESH

Two beets chopped

One large pear

Two large carrots

One cup fresh pineapple

TOMATO JUICING BENEFITS

Tomato juice offers essential vitamins such as Vitamin A, K, and B vitamins which are required for daily function. Tomato juice also contains levels of magnesium, iron, and phosphorous. It contains many health benefits that numerous fruits and vegetables don't usually obtain. The water and vitamins within tomatoes obtain a healthy colon and protect against colon cancer. Tomatoes nutrients also protect against prostate cancer, pancreatic cancer, cervical cancer, mouth cancer, and heart disease. These wonderful fruits obtain anti-inflammatory properties which is beneficial to many different areas within our bodies. Eating tomatoes increases Vitamin C levels within our blood, leading to reduction or disappearance in anxiety and stress. Because tomatoes contain high levels of Vitamin K, they are known to promote positive bone health and partner with the intake of calcium as vitamin K helps obtain calcium within the bones. Vitamin K is also known to improve the health of your eyes and your eyesight, and can benefit the healthiness of your skin and hair. Adding tomato juice to your daily diet can promote the inner and outer beauty of our wonderful bodies!

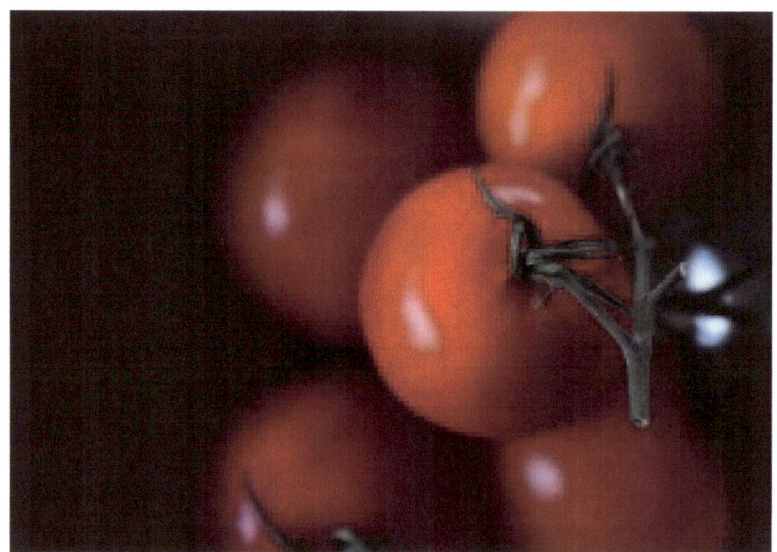

Tomato Juicing Recipes

TOMATO TANGO

Four tomatoes

½ red pepper

Three large carrots

Two stalks of celery

One cup spinach

One clove fresh garlic

½ large lemon

Dash of salt and pepper

RED SPICE

Four large tomatoes

Three stalks celery

¼ teaspoon oregano

¼ teaspoon fresh parsley

SWEET SENSATION

Three large tomatoes

One small sweet potato

Three medium carrots

One cucumber

One large lemon

One large lime

SUNRISE

Two large tomatoes

Two stalks celery

Two large carrots

½ cup pineapple

½ large lime

SWEET PEPPER SURPRISE

Three large tomatoes

One large red pepper

One large yellow pepper

Two stalks celery

Two large carrots

RED BLAST

Four large tomatoes

Two cups fresh strawberries

KICKIN JUICE

Four large tomatoes

Two green onion sticks

½ green pepper

Two large carrots

Two stalks celery

Handful cilantro

One large lemon

SWEET AND SOUR SUNRISE

Three large tomatoes

Four large carrots

Two stalks celery

One cup fresh pineapple chunks

Two large lemons

VEGGY BLAST

Four large tomatoes

Five large carrots

Two stalks kale

Two stalks celery

Two medium lemons

SUMMER SIDEKICK

Three large tomatoes

Three stalks celery

½ yellow pepper

½ red pepper

Handful cilantro

BERRY JUICING BENEFITS

These berry juicing recipes contain a variety of berries including strawberries, blueberries, blackberries, and raspberries. All of these berries contain health benefits that differ from the others.

Strawberries have numerous benefits while they remain low in calories. They obtain antioxidants, anti-cancer nutrients such as Vitamin C and folate, and they also boost the immune system. Strawberry juice is also used as a natural teeth whitener and helps create beautiful skin.

Blueberries are known as one of the world's super foods, due to their high nutritional value per small portion. They are extremely high in Vitamin A, C, and E, resulting in their antioxidant properties that protect our body cells.

Blackberries and raspberries are filled with antioxidants, hence the extremely dark vibrant color they possess. They are low in calories and fat free while obtaining high levels of nutrients for our bodies. Blackberry juice and raspberry juice is extremely beneficial for heart health as it protects and replenishes tissues that have occurred damage due to oxidants in the body. Studies show that blackberries and raspberries may increase motor and cognitive skills that decrease as you get older and inquire health issues. Blackberry juice and raspberry juice can also prevent the decline of motor and cognitive skills if it is incorporated in your daily diet at a relatively young age.

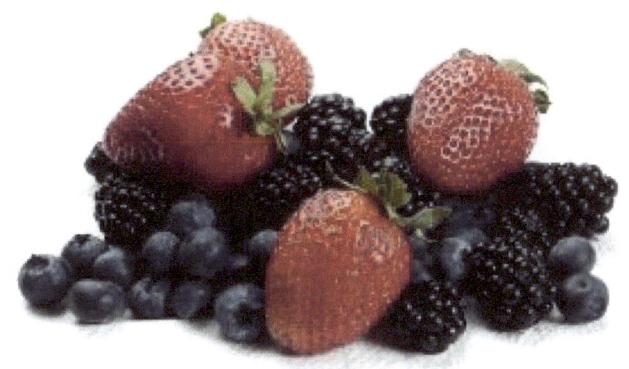

Berry Juicing Recipes

BERRY BLAST

15 strawberries

Two cups fresh blueberries

Two cups spinach

TROPICAL BERRY JUICE

15 large strawberries

One cup fresh pineapple

Two medium oranges

One stalk celery

One stalk kale

PURPLE PARADISE

Two cups purple grapes

Two cups fresh blackberries

One cup spinach

One large lemon

BERRY SCRUMPTIOUS

One large granny smith apple

Two cups fresh blueberries

One cup blackberries

One cup spinach

One large lime

SWEET CITRUS JUICE

One sweet potato- cooked and cooled

Two cups fresh pineapple

One large lime

½ stick lemon grass

DETOXIFYING BERRY BLAST

One red ruby grapefruit

Two cups fresh strawberries

Two cups blackberries

One large lemon

TROPICAL TANG

One cup fresh pineapple

Two cups blackberries

One large pear

Two kiwifruit

SMART TART

One large pear

Two cups blackberries

One cup raspberries

One cup fresh pineapple chunks

SWEET SMOOTH BLEND

Two cups fresh strawberries

One large peach

One cup fresh pineapples

One cup blueberries

TROPICAL WATERS

One cup banana puree

Two cup raspberries

One large fresh mango

One cup blueberries

FINAL THOUGHTS

Juicing fruits are vegetables have a positive effect on your overall health and lifestyle. Take charge by incorporating these delicious healthy juicing blends into your daily diet instead of avoiding various fruits and vegetables. This book is a reference book; you can continuously refer to the health benefits of these various fruits and vegetables and choose a different juice blend each day. I encourage you to write a food journal consisting of the whole foods and juicing blend you ingest. Within this journal, describe how you feel at the end of each day and see if the addition of fresh juice makes a positive difference in your life. If you find yourself having a negative effect from a specific juice recipe, avoid ingesting that specific juice blend in the future. Some individuals enjoy different types of flavors than other individuals, and our bodies execute that same aspect when it comes to juicing mixtures. Remember to change the type of juice blend you drink each day so you are able to receive all the health benefits that these delicious refreshing juices have to offer.

Thank you so much for purchasing this juicing recipe book and I hope you enjoy these fresh juicing recipes as much as I do! If you could, please leave a review for my book. Each review means a great deal to me. It gives me valuable feedback to improve my writing and future books for you.

To Your Health,

Jamie Fox

www.ingramcontent.com/pod-product-compliance
Lightning Source LLC
Chambersburg PA
CBHW041501280526
45792CB00004B/1088